I0701895

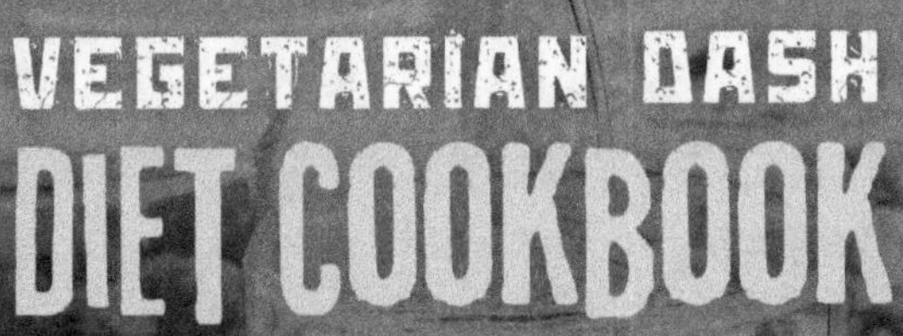

VEGETARIAN DASH
DIET COOKBOOK
Explore Low Sodium and Low Fat Recipes
for Lower Blood Pressure, Reduced Heart
Disease, and Lasting Health Benefits.
ELIZABETH V. CARRINGTON

Thanks for Purchasing My Book!

Here is your reward!

Thank you immensely for choosing my book! To express my gratitude, I've created a special perk for you. Should you encounter any challenges or have questions about a recipe – whether it's about tweaking ingredients or ensuring a flawless outcome – feel free to reach out. Your satisfaction is my priority. Simply send an email to **elizabethcarringtoncooks@gmail.com**, detailing your query, and I'll promptly provide the solution you're looking for. Consider this my way of extending thanks and supporting you on your dietary journey.

Don't hesitate to take advantage of this offer. Your culinary success matters, and I'm here to help.

Happy cooking!

Table Of Contents

INTRODUCTION

I met Mary in the hospital where my grandma was admitted. We were in the same ward so we talked for a long time and she will always be on the lookout for me every day I visit. I learned she has been diagnosed with hypertension. She is 45 and her sons were not in town then. They only sent money to her for her medical checkup. She said I would not have met her in the hospital if she had followed the doctor's directives for not taking excess sodium and a lot of fat. However, she would not listen because she loved those things dearly.

I had not introduced myself then so we were just talking about our personal experiences with life challenges. That is when I told her that my grandma was in her condition three years back but I helped her get over it. She managed hypertension through my dietary recommendations from the doctor's advice. Therefore, I went into deep research following the best chefs, and studying the effect of some food combinations on disease management. That was how I structured a meal plan for my grandma which she followed and maintained normal health.

Mary was so happy hearing that I helped my grandma so she pleaded for the recipes too. I was hesitant to give her the recipe book because I did not know if her house help could prepare the dishes. Nevertheless, on second thought, I decided to give her one when I next visited the hospital.

The next day, I handed over the recipe book to her with some guidelines on the preparation methods for the seemingly hard to prepare dishes. "The best gift I have ever received from people this year so far is this book," she said. I looked at her, laughed, and assured her she would be fine if she strictly followed it. The last time we talked she sounded so lovely over the phone and told me her blood pressure was coming down to normal level. Therefore, she was sure she had a solution to her problem.

I know the stress of trying to figure out your dishes all by yourself. I know the challenges of going back to the hospital are worse than when you first visited. I know how hard it can be to keep taking those medications even when you do not like taking them or you do not even have the financial muscle to foot the bills. That is why I have decided to hand over the same recipe book to you right now, though with newly discovered dishes that will help you get the better health you have ever desired. I need you to assure me you will stick to it and get the best result. You have to believe it will work for you too as you work towards better health.

Now get ready to cook that delicacy that not only nourishes your body but helps you get better in health challenges. I included a five-week meal plan at the end of this book so you can easily decide on what to cook for breakfast, lunch, and dinner with some tasty snacks and desserts to go down with the main dishes.

What is Hypertension

High blood pressure, also known as hypertension, refers to blood pressure levels above the normal range. Fluctuations in blood pressure occur throughout the day based on activities, and consistent readings above normal may lead to a diagnosis of hypertension. The elevated blood pressure poses an increased risk of various health issues, including heart disease, heart attack, and stroke.

Diagnosis and treatment decisions for high blood pressure are made by the health care team through an evaluation of systolic and diastolic blood pressure levels, comparing them to specific guidelines. These guidelines may vary among health care professionals:
Some practitioners diagnose high blood pressure if readings consistently register at 140/90 mm Hg or higher. Others identify hypertension when readings consistently measure 130/80 mm Hg or higher.

Hypertension Leads to Other Health Issues

High blood pressure can adversely impact vital organs such as the heart, brain, kidneys, and eyes, posing significant health risks. It can impair arterial elasticity, reducing blood and oxygen flow to the heart and contributing to conditions like heart disease. The consequences may include chest pain (angina), heart attacks resulting from blocked blood supply, and heart failure, where the heart cannot pump sufficient blood to other organs.

In the case of the brain, high blood pressure can lead to burst or blocked arteries, causing strokes. Stroke-induced brain cell death due to inadequate oxygen can result in severe disabilities and, in some instances, prove fatal. Additionally, high blood pressure, particularly in midlife, is associated with diminished cognitive function and an increased risk of dementia later in life.

The encouraging news is that, in most instances, proactive management of blood pressure can mitigate the risk of serious health issues. Lifestyle changes play a crucial role, and individuals can discuss the following strategies with their healthcare team:

- ❖ Engaging in a minimum of 150 minutes of physical activity per week (approximately 30 minutes daily for five days).
- ❖ Abstaining from smoking.
- ❖ **Adopting a healthy diet, which includes limiting sodium (salt) and alcohol intake**.
- ❖ Maintaining a healthy weight.
- ❖ Effectively managing stress.

These lifestyle modifications empower individuals to either lower their elevated blood pressure into a healthy range or sustain healthy blood pressure levels.

Causes of Hypertension

High blood pressure often lacks a definitive cause, with various factors contributing to an increased risk. Individuals may find themselves more susceptible if they:

- ❖ Carry excess weight
- ❖ Consume excessive salt while neglecting fruits and vegetables
- ❖ Lead a sedentary lifestyle
- ❖ Engage in excessive alcohol, coffee, or caffeine-based drink consumption

- ❖ Smoke

- ❖ Experience heightened stress levels

- ❖ Surpass the age of 65

- ❖ Possess a family history of high blood pressure

- ❖ Reside in economically deprived areas

Adopting healthier lifestyle choices can potentially mitigate the likelihood of developing high blood pressure and assist in lowering existing elevated blood pressure. Notably, approximately 1 in 10 cases of high blood pressure stem from underlying health conditions or specific medications. Contributing health conditions encompass:

- ❖ Kidney disease

- ❖ Diabetes

- ❖ Hormonal imbalances, such as underactive or overactive thyroid, Cushing's syndrome, acromegaly, elevated aldosterone levels (hyperaldosteronism), and pheochromocytoma

- ❖ Lupus, an autoimmune disorder targeting various body parts

- ❖ Scleroderma, a condition resulting in thickened skin and potential organ and blood vessel complications
- ❖ Prolonged kidney infections
- ❖ Sleep apnea, characterized by the relaxation and narrowing of throat walls during sleep, disrupting normal breathing.
- ❖ Glomerulonephritis, involving damage to the tiny filters within the kidneys
- ❖ Arterial narrowing supplying the kidneys

Certain medications can also contribute to increased blood pressure, including:

- ❖ Steroids
- ❖ Recreational drugs such as cocaine and amphetamines.
- ❖ Non-steroidal anti-inflammatory drugs (NSAIDs) like ibuprofen, aspirin, and naproxen
- ❖ Herbal remedies, particularly those containing liquorice
- ❖ Contraceptive pills
- ❖ Specific cough and cold remedies

❖ Selective serotonin-noradrenaline reuptake inhibitor (SSNRI) antidepressants like venlafaxine.

It's worth noting that discontinuing the use of these medications or substances may lead to a normalization of blood pressure in such cases.

BREAKFAST

Even though we only get around eight hours of sleep each night, breakfast is often cited as the most significant meal of the day. As a result, there are many times when the stomach is empty of both food and liquids. For this reason, it makes perfect sense that eating breakfast will provide us with the energy we need to go through the day and regain our strength.

1. Avocado Toast And With Tomato

Ten minutes for cooking

Ingredients (two servings' worth):

- ❖ Cloves of garlic
- ❖ Newly picked thyme
- ❖ Cherry tomatoes
- ❖ Extra virgin olive oil
- ❖ Slices of bread

❖ Lemon

❖ Parsley

❖ Avocados

❖ Recently ground black pepper

❖ Salt

Guidelines

❖ Cut the cloves of garlic, Add the cherry tomatoes, garlic, and fresh thyme to the baking dish. The tomatoes should be above the garlic.

❖ After spooning the olive oil over the tomatoes, toss them to ensure they are uniformly covered, either with your hands or a big spoon.

❖ After the tomatoes begin to wrinkle and some burst in the baking pan, roast them for 15 to 20 minutes. When the roasted tomatoes have cooled to room temperature, remove the baking dish from the oven.

❖ Toast the bread pieces and drizzle with the olive oil from the tomato. Put it away.

❖ Keep the pan's olive oil aside. This oil will be used to season the avocado and to drizzle over the bread. It tastes wonderfully like garlic. I prefer to eat it simply with bread because it's that delicious.

❖ Prepare the other ingredients before you begin preparing the avocado combination. Chop the parsley finely and juice the lemon.

❖ Cut the avocados in half and chop them up into a basin. Add the salt, lemon juice, tomato olive oil, and chopped parsley.

❖ Mash the ingredients and avocado together. After tasting, adjust the amount of salt, lemon juice, and tomato olive oil.

❖ Top each slice with a little bit of the mashed avocado. Top each slice with a few of the roasted tomatoes. Next, add the chopped basil or parsley.

❖ Over the avocado toast, drizzle a little more of the tomato olive oil. Add a dash of salt and freshly ground black pepper on top. The avocado mixture will oxidize and begin to turn brown, so serve the avocado toast immediately.

2. Quinoa Breakfast Bowl

Ingredients

- ❖ Quinoa: This is one of the important components, therefore we're going to start with 2 cups of uncooked quinoa. This dish is a good way to use up leftover quinoa for a quick breakfast. However, you may easily create more if you don't have any leftovers on hand.

- ❖ Garlic: I adore fresh garlic, but if you don't feel like peeling garlic in the morning, garlic powder is a good choice.

- ❖ Bell pepper: we selected red pepper for color, but any bell pepper would work.

- ❖ Spinach: wilt this down for an almost undetectable component that is packed in iron and fiber.

- ❖ Cherry tomatoes: a fresh crisp tomato adds color and taste to these bowls.

- ❖ Avocado: fill out the dish with healthy fats (and additional fiber!).

- ❖ Eggs: the jammy eggs are show-stoppers. They look fantastic and taste much better.

Guidelines

- Quinoa: prepare the quinoa according to the package instructions if you haven't already. For additional flavor, boil your quinoa in veggie broth. Cooking the quinoa ahead of time speeds this dish up even further.

- Saute the veggies: heat olive oil in a medium skillet over medium-high heat. Add the garlic and sauté for 30 seconds then add the red pepper and cook for 1-2 minutes, until tender. Add another tablespoon of olive oil then add the spinach and heat, turning regularly, until the spinach has wilted, 2-3 minutes.

- Mix the quinoa and vegetables: Add the cooked quinoa and salt to the skillet with the veggies and mix thoroughly.

- Jammy eggs: boil the eggs for 6 ½ minutes then move to an ice bath. See the section above or the recipe card for further instructions.

- Assemble: Add the quinoa mixture to a serving dish and top with avocado, sliced tomatoes, and cooked eggs. Sprinkle with extra salt, everything bagel seasoning, hemp seeds, or more salt, if desired

3. Black Bean Breakfast Bowl

Ten minutes for preparation

5 minutes to cook

15 minutes in total

Yield: 2; Servings: 2.

Ingredients

- ❖ Two tsp olive oil
- ❖ Four beaten eggs
- ❖ One fifteen-ounce can of rinsed and drained black beans
- ❖ Halved and sliced avocado;
- ❖ ¼ cup salsa;
- ❖ To taste, add salt and ground black pepper

Guidelines

- ❖ In a small pan set over medium heat, warm the olive oil. For three to five minutes, cook and whisk eggs until they are set.
- ❖ Put black beans in a dish that is safe to microwave. Cook in the microwave on High for 1 minute, or until thoroughly cooked.

- ❖ Spoon two bowls of warmed black beans over each other.
- ❖ Add salsa, avocado, and scrambled eggs to the top of each bowl. Sprinkle it with a little salt and black pepper.

Facts about Nutrition (per serving)

625 Calories, 28g protein, 47g carbs, and 39g fat

4. Greek Yogurt Parfait

Ingredients

- ❖ Half a cup of raw blueberries
- ❖ ½ cup of freshly sliced strawberries
- ❖ One tsp of white sugar, if desired
- ❖ 6 tablespoons granola, or as required
- ❖ 1 (6 ounces) carton of nonfat vanilla Greek yogurt
- ❖ One tsp lemon zest

Guidelines

- ❖ Fill a small basin with strawberries and blueberries.
- ❖ Dredge in sugar and toss to coat the berries.

- ❖ Fill two parfait glasses with two teaspoons of granola. Top with 2 tablespoons of yogurt and 1/2 teaspoon of lemon zest.
- ❖ Add a third of the berries on top. Once the parfait glasses are filled, continue layering.

Facts about Nutrition (per serving)

264 Calories, 26g Carbs, 9g Protein, and 14g Fat

5. Berry and nut oatmeal

Ingredients:

- ❖ 3/4 cup organic old-fashioned oats
- ❖ 1/2 cup water and 2 tablespoons ground flaxseeds
- ❖ One tablespoon of chia seeds
- ❖ One cup organic berries and 1/4 teaspoon salt I often use frozen
- ❖ 1/4 cup mixed nuts or walnuts

Guidelines

- ❖ Heat 1 1/2 cups of water, oatmeal, chia seeds, crushed flax, and salt until they boil.
- ❖ Reduce the heat and let the oatmeal simmer for 7 to 10 minutes, or until the water has evaporated and it becomes tender.
- ❖ Slice berries into small pieces.
- ❖ Serve oatmeal with soy yogurt or nut milk on top, topped with the nuts and berries.

6. Whole wheat pancakes

Preparation Time: 10 mins

Cooking Time: 20 mins

Total Time: 30 mins

Servings: 4

Ingredients

- ❖ 2 cups whole wheat flour
- ❖ 2 tablespoons white sugar
- ❖ 2 teaspoons baking powder
- ❖ ½ teaspoon baking soda
- ❖ ½ teaspoon sal

- ❖ 2 ¼ cups buttermilk

- ❖ 2 large eggs

- ❖ 4 tablespoons vegetable oil, divided

Guidelines

- ❖ Whisk flour, sugar, baking powder, baking soda, and salt together in a bowl.

- ❖ Whisk buttermilk, eggs, and 3 tablespoons oil together in a separate bowl until well combined. Pour wet ingredients into dry ingredients and stir until just combined; batter may seem a bit thick.

- ❖ Heat remaining 1 tablespoon oil in a cast iron skillet over medium-low heat for 5 minutes.

- ❖ Working in batches, pour 1/3 cup of batter for each pancake into the hot skillet. Spread batter into circles with a spoon; cook until browned on the bottom and bubbles appear on top, 1 1/2 to 2 minutes. Flip and cook until set in the middle and browned on the other side, about 2 more minutes.

Nutrition Facts (per serving)
410 Calories, 15g Fat, 57g Carbs, 16g Protein.

7. Veggies Omelette

Servings: One serving

358 CALORIES

SETUP TIME: ten minutes

Cooking time: ten minutes

Twenty minutes in total

Ingredients:

- ❖ One-third cup of finely chopped red onions and one tablespoon of olive oil
- ❖ ¼ cup of red peppers chopped finely
- ❖ Sliced mushrooms, ¼ cup
- ❖ One cup of newly harvested baby spinach
- ❖ To taste, add salt and pepper.
- ❖ two to three eggs
- ❖ One tablespoon of water
- ❖ Two tablespoons of cheddar cheese, shredded
- ❖ To serve, fresh parsley

Guidelines

- ❖ In an 8- or 10-inch nonstick pan, heat the olive oil over medium heat. Cook the red onions, red peppers, and mushrooms for three to five minutes, or until they are crisp-tender. After adding the spinach, simmer for another minute or so, or until the spinach wilts. After transferring the veggies to a small dish, clean the pan.

❖ In a small dish, crack and beat eggs with water. Transfer the egg mixture to the same pan. Using a spatula, carefully push the cooked parts into the middle of the pan as the eggs start to set around the skillet's edge. To let raw eggs spill into voids, tilt and rotate the pan.

❖ Add the cooked veggies to half of the omelet and sprinkle the cheddar cheese on top when the eggs are nearly set. After putting a spatula underneath the empty part, fold it over.

❖ Transfer to a dish with care from the skillet. Serve right away, garnished with fresh parsley and seasoned with salt and pepper.

8 Sweet Potato and Black Bean Breakfast Burrito

Twenty minutes for preparation

Cooking Time: 60 minutes

One hour thirty minutes in total

Yield: 4 servings; Servings: 4.

Ingredients

- ❖ Two pounds of peeled and cubed orange-fleshed sweet potatoes
- ❖ Half a teaspoon of dried chipotle pepper, ground
- ❖ Half a teaspoon of salt
- ❖ Two tsp olive oil, separated
- ❖ One chopped onion and four minced garlic cloves
- ❖ One jalapeño pepper, cut; one red bell pepper, chopped
- ❖ two teaspoons of ancho chili powder, or to taste
- ❖ One tablespoon of cumin powder
- ❖ One-half tsp dried oregano
- ❖ One (28-oz) can of chopped tomatoes
- ❖ One cup of water, or to your taste
- ❖ One spoonful of cornmeal
- ❖ 1 tsp salt, or more to taste

- ❖ One tsp white sugar

- ❖ 1 tsp powdered unsweetened cocoa

- ❖ 2 (fifteen-ounce) cans of rinsed and drained black beans

- ❖ One cayenne pepper pinch, or according to taste

- ❖ ½ cup of sour cream, optionally garnished

- ❖ For garnish, cut ¼ cup of fresh cilantro (optional).

Guidelines

- ❖ First, heat the oven to 400 degrees Fahrenheit (200 degrees Celsius). Line a baking pan with silicone mats or parchment paper.

- ❖ In a large bowl, combine the sweet potatoes, chipotle pepper, 1/2 teaspoon salt, and 1 tablespoon olive oil to coat. Arrange sweet potatoes in a single layer on the baking sheet that has been preheated.

- ❖ Roast the sweet potatoes for 20 to 25 minutes, or until the exterior is crispy and the center is soft. Once at room temperature, let it cool.

- ❖ In a large saucepan or Dutch oven over medium heat, cook and mix the remaining 1 tablespoon olive oil, onion, garlic, red bell pepper, jalapeño pepper, ancho chile powder, cumin, and dried oregano. Allow onion to soften and stir for about five minutes.

❖ Add water and tomatoes to the onion mixture and cook. Add sugar, cocoa powder, cornmeal, and one teaspoon of salt. Bring to a boil while stirring continuously. On low heat boil for 30 minutes.

❖ Incorporate the cooled sweet potatoes and black beans into the onion-tomato mixture. Add more water to the mixture if it's too thick.

❖ Simmer for 15 minutes or until well heated. To taste, add cayenne and salt for seasoning. Garnish with sour cream and cilantro and serve.

Facts about Nutrition (per serving)
600 Calorie
21g Protein, 101g Carbs, and 15g Fat

9. Spinach and Feta Omelet

Preparation time: 10 minutes.

5 minutes to cook

15 minutes in total

Servings: One; Yield: One

Ingredients for cooking spray

* Three egg whites, to taste, with salt and powdered black pepper
* ¼ cup of freshly chopped spinach, or more to taste
* Two tablespoons of feta cheese crumbles and six sliced cherry tomatoes

Guidelines

* Apply cooking spray to a skillet and heat it over medium heat.
* In a bowl, whisk together egg whites, salt, and pepper. After adding the egg mixture to the hot pan and swirling it around until the eggs cover the whole bottom, cook for one to two minutes.

❖ Place feta cheese, tomatoes, and spinach in the center of the eggs. Cook for a further two to three minutes, or until the edges of the eggs start to curl.

❖ Using a spatula, remove the omelet from the pan and fold it in half. Cook for two to three minutes, or until the cheese has melted.

10. Mango-Chia Seed Pudding

Ingredients:

- ❖ 1 cup Greek yogurt, reduced fat
- ❖ Half a cup of unprocessed honey
- ❖ Four tsp matcha tea powder (like the kind made by Full Leaf Tea Company)
- ❖ One tsp vanilla essence
- ❖ One cup of coconut milk without sugar
- ❖ half a cup of chia seeds
- ❖ two cups of chunky mango

Guidelines

- ❖ In a dish, whisk together yogurt, honey, matcha powder, and vanilla extract. Whisk in chia seeds and slowly stir in coconut milk.
- ❖ Refrigerate the yogurt mixture for at least 4 hours or overnight, or until it thickens, Cover with plastic wrap.
- ❖ Put the pieces of mango into a blender and process until smooth.

❖ Transfer the yogurt mixture into four glasses or bowls for serving, and then equally top with mango puree.

Facts about Nutrition (per serving)

256 Calories

8g Protein, 25g Carbs, and 16g Fat

11. Pineapple and Cottage Cheese Bowl

Ingredients

- ❖ One-fourth cup of natural yogurt or cottage cheese
- ❖ Half a cup of pineapple dice
- ❖ Two teaspoons of seeds from pomegranates
- ❖ One tablespoon of coconut grated
- ❖ One tablespoon of almonds, slivered

Guidelines

- ❖ Get the pineapple ready by thoroughly draining it through a strainer. Cut the pineapple chunks into bite-sized pieces if they are too big. Pineapple crushed is OK as well; just be sure to drain it well before using. If you're using fresh fruit, begin by cutting and peeling it.

- ❖ Use a food processor or blender to whip the cheese (1,2). See our recipe for Whipped Cottage Cheese for full directions.

- ❖ Alternatively, don't alter the cottage cheese. Although we like its whipped smoothness, real lumpy, curd-like cheese is equally delicious; it just comes down to taste choice.

12. Overnight Oats with Blueberries and Almonds

Five minutes for preparation

Five minutes in total

One serving

Ingredients

- ❖ ½ cup of rolled oats
- ❖ A quarter cup of almond milk
- ❖ Two tablespoons of almond butter
- ❖ ½ teaspoon each of ground cinnamon and vanilla extract
- ❖ One cup of split frozen highbush blueberries
- ❖ One tablespoon of almond slices, roasted

Guidelines

- ❖ Oats, almond butter, almond milk, vanilla, and cinnamon should all be combined in a mason jar.
- ❖ Add ½ cup blueberries and stir.
- ❖ Add the sliced almonds and the remaining ½ cup blueberries on top.

❖ Shut up. Chill for four hours or overnight.

LUNCH

1. Mediterranean Chickpea Salad

15 minutes for preparation

Three hours extra

Three hours in total fifteen minutes

Yield: 4 servings; Servings: 4.

Ingredients

- ❖ 1 (15-ounce) can of washed and drained garbanzo beans, or chickpeas
- ❖ ½ cup sun-dried tomatoes packed with oil drained, and sliced into strips
- ❖ One cup of feta cheese, crumbled
- ❖ One sliced red onion and two minced garlic cloves
- ❖ One tablespoon of freshly cut cilantro
- ❖ Two tsp olive oil
- ❖ Two tsp lemon juice
- ❖ Salt according to taste

- ❖ Combine the feta cheese, sun-dried tomatoes, onion, garlic, cilantro, and garbanzo beans in a bowl.
- ❖ Mix the olive oil, lemon juice, and salt in another dish and drizzle it over the salad.
- ❖ When serving, refrigerate for a minimum of three hours.

Facts about Nutrition (per serving)

354 Calories

14g Protein, 25g Carbs, and 23g Fat

2. Fried rice with cauliflower:

2. Cauliflower Fried Rice:

15 minutes for preparation

Cooking Duration: 30 minutes

45 minutes in total

Yield: 6 servings; Servings: 6.

Ingredients

- ❖ Split 2 cups frozen peas

- ❖ ½ cup water

- ❖ ¼ cup sesame oil.

- ❖ Four glasses of Cubed Pork Loin

- ❖ Six thinly sliced green onions

- ❖ one big carrot diced

- ❖ Two minced garlic cloves

- ❖ 20 ounces of cauliflower, shredded

- ❖ Six tsp soy sauce

- ❖ two beaten eggs

Guidelines

- ❖ Combine the peas and water in a saucepan; stir and bring to a boil. Then, decrease the heat to medium-low and continue cooking and stirring for 5 minutes or until the peas are soft and cooked through. Remove and dispose of water.

- ❖ In a wok, heat two tablespoons of sesame oil over medium-high heat. Pork should be cooked thoroughly and gently browned on both sides after 7 to 10 minutes of cooking and stirring in hot oil. Place the meat onto a platter.

❖ Warm up the last two teaspoons of sesame oil. Heat oil and saute green onions, carrot, and garlic until they become somewhat tender, approximately 5 minutes. After adding the cauliflower, simmer and toss it for 4 to 5 minutes, or until it has a firm bite but is still soft.

❖ Add the pork, peas, and soy sauce to the cauliflower mixture and stir-fry for 3 to 5 minutes, or until the mixture is hot and starting to brown.

❖ Transfer the pork cauliflower combination to one side of the pan and cover the empty side with beaten eggs. After 3 to 5 minutes of scrambling, add the cooked eggs to the pork cauliflower mixture, being sure to break up any big lumps.

Facts about Nutrition (per serving)

367 Calorie

33g Protein, 16g Carbs, and 19g Fat

3. Chickpea and Spinach Quesadilla

Ingredients

- 19 oz can of white beans, drained and rinsed
- 3 ounces of chopped spinach (see note 2
- One teaspoon each of ground coriander and cumin
- One-half teaspoon of salt
- ¾ cup of crumbled feta cheese
- One-third cup of shredded mozzarella
- Five big or 12-inch tortillas

Guidelines

- Thaw and squeeze out excess moisture if the spinach is frozen.
- Use a fork or potato masher to mash the white beans in a big basin.
- Add the salt, cumin, coriander, and spinach and stir. After the spinach has somewhat wilted, stir or mash it and add in the feta cheese.
- Turn up the heat to medium in a big pan. Cook two quesadillas at a time in the pan after spraying with oil.

❖ Spoon out ½ cup of the filling made of white beans and spinach, and then top with ¼ cup of cheese. After folding the tortilla over, firmly push it down.

❖ Cook until brown and crispy, about 3 minutes on each side.

Information on Nutrition

One quesadilla is served, with 396 kcal, 37 g of carbohydrates, 19 g of protein, and 20 g of fat.

11g of saturated fat, 54 mg of cholesterol, 1030 mg of sodium, 5 g of fiber, and 2 g of sugar

4. Vegan Coconut-Lentil Curry with Sweet Potatoes

15 minutes for preparation

Cooking Time: 55 Minutes

One hour and ten minutes total

Yield: 6 servings; Servings: 6.

Ingredients

❖ 2 tablespoons coconut oil and 3 cups vegetable broth.

* one chopped medium yellow onion

* Two teaspoons of masala garam

* Two tsp finely chopped garlic, split

* One 28-oz can of crushed tomatoes

* 1/4 cup finely chopped fresh ginger root and 1/4 cup turmeric

* Two tsp sea salt and one cup of dry lentils

* Cubed one medium sweet potato

* one-tsp cayenne pepper, or more to taste

* One fifteen-ounce container of shaken coconut milk

* Three cups cooked basmati rice and one spoonful of freshly chopped cilantro

Guidelines

* In a medium saucepan, bring 3 cups of vegetable broth to a boil.

* In the meantime, bring a big saucepan of coconut oil to a boil over medium-high heat. Add onion and sauté for approximately 5 minutes, or until tender and transparent.

* Add the spices for tikka masala, stir, and cook for one minute. Add the garlic and simmer for about a

minute, or until fragrant but not burned. Add the salt, turmeric, ginger, and tomatoes. Stir-fry for five minutes.

❖ Stir in the sweet potato, lentils, cayenne, and spicy vegetable broth. Heat to a boil over a medium-high flame. After the sweet potato and lentils are well cooked, which should take approximately 40 minutes, reduce heat, cover, and simmer, stirring often to avoid sticking.

❖ Stir in coconut milk after adding it. Heat through to a simmer. Take off the heat and serve with rice and cilantro on top.

Facts about Nutrition (per serving)

504 Calories

16g Protein, 67g Carbs, and 21g Fat

Vegetarian sushi bowl

Preparation time: 45 minutes.

15 minutes for cooking

Extra Time: Ten Minutes

One hour and ten minutes total

4 servings; 4 sushi rolls are produced.

Ingredients

- ❖ 1 ½ cups uncooked white short-grain rice
- ❖ 1/2 cup red wine vinegar and 1 ½ cups water
- ❖ Two tsp white sugar
- ❖ One tsp salt
- ❖ ½ avocado, finely cut, pitted and peeled
- ❖ one tsp lemon juice
- ❖ 1/4 cup sesame seeds, or as required; 1 cup peeled, seeded, and matchstick-cut cucumber
- ❖ Cut a ½ green bell pepper into matchsticks after the seeds are removed.
- ❖ ½ cup chopped matchstick-sized zucchini

Guidelines

- ❖ In a saucepan, combine rice and water; heat to a boil, then immediately lower the heat. After approximately 15 minutes, or until the water is absorbed, cook the rice with a cover that fits tightly. After turning off the heat, cover the rice and let it stand for ten minutes.

* In a basin, stir together red wine vinegar, sugar, and salt until sugar is dissolved. After using a fork to fluff the rice, move it into a large bowl, add the vinegar mixture, and toss to coat the rice.

* After the rice is spread out onto a large piece of parchment paper, fan it until it cools. Wrap rice with wet paper towels.

* In a bowl, drizzle avocado slices with lemon juice.

* Drizzle a sushi mat with a thin coating of sesame seeds. Take roughly a half-cup of the chilled rice and spread it evenly on the sushi mat.

* Arrange 1/4 of the bell pepper, zucchini, cucumber, avocado slices, and zucchini in a line along the center of the rice.

* Resolve the sushi mat's edge, fold the bottom edge up to enclose the filling, and roll the sushi firmly into a thick cylinder.

* When the sushi is rolled, place it within the mat and give it a little press to firmly compact it.

- ❖ To make four rolls, repeat with the remaining ingredients. Rolls should be placed on a serving platter, cut into six or eight pieces each, and then covered with wet paper towels until it's ready to serve.

Facts about Nutrition (per serving)

385 Calorie, 70g Carbs, 9g Fat, and 8g Protein

6. Hummus and Roasted Vegetable Preparation

Time: Ten minutes

25 minutes for cooking

35 minutes total

Six wraps are served.

194 kcal of calories

- ❖ Six wholemeal tortilla wrappers (whole wheat wrappers) are needed.
- ❖ One medium-sized sweet potato
- ❖ One red pepper
- ❖ One zucchini

❖ Two tablespoons of paste made with harissa

❖ Six tsp hummus and one cup of fresh baby spinach

Guidelines

❖ Cut the sweet potato, red pepper, and zucchini into tiny cubes. Add the harissa paste and stir well.

❖ Roast for 20 to 25 minutes at 200 degrees Celsius (390 degrees Fahrenheit).

❖ Spread a spoonful of hummus on a tortilla wrap. Top with roasted vegetables and fresh baby spinach.

❖ Make sure the edges are securely secured when you wrap it.

Facts About Nutrition

194 kcal of calories, 32g of carbohydrates, 6g of protein, 4g of fat, 1g of saturated fat, 429 mg of sodium, 280 mg of potassium, 5g of fiber, 5g of sugar, 4265 IU of vitamin A, 33.9 mg of vitamin C, 104 mg of calcium, and 2 mg of iron.

7. Vegetable and Lentil Soup

Twenty minutes for preparation

1 hour 30 minutes for cooking

Extra Time: One Hour and Ten Minutes

Three hours in total

Yield: 6 to 1 cup servings; 6 serves

Ingredients:

* ½ cup lentils, either red or green
* One cup of chopped onion, one chopped celery stalk, and two cups of shredded cabbage
* One 28-oz can of chopped whole peeled tomatoes and two cups of chicken broth
* three sliced carrots, one smashed garlic clove
* ½ teaspoon crushed black pepper, ¼ teaspoon white sugar, and one teaspoon salt
* One-half teaspoon of dried basil
* ½ teaspoon curry powder; ½ teaspoon dried thyme

Guidelines

* Pour water into a stock pot or Dutch oven until the lentils are twice as deep as the container. After bringing it to a boil, reduce heat, and simmer for

around fifteen minutes. Rinse and drain the lentils, then put them back in the saucepan.

❖ Toss in the onion, celery, cabbage, tomatoes, chicken stock, carrots, and garlic. Season with the curry, sugar, salt, and pepper.

❖ Simmer for one and a half to two hours, or until the desired level of tenderness is reached.

❖ In a slow cooker, combine ingredients; simmer on Low for 8 to 10 hours, or on High for approximately 4 hours, or until veggies are cooked and lentils are broken down.

Facts about Nutrition (per serving)

112 energy, 22g Carbs, 1g Fat, and 6g Protein

8. Caprese salad with Balsamic glaze

Each serving quantity (6 serves)

Ingredients

❖ 3 vine-ripened or heirloom tomatoes, sliced into ¼-inch pieces

- ❖ One pound of fresh mozzarella cut into ¼-inch slices (pre-sliced is fine) and combined with ½ teaspoon sugar and ½ teaspoon salt.
- ❖ freshly ground peppercorns, according to taste.
- ❖ Olive oil that is extra virgin, to drizzle
- ❖ Store-bought balsamic glaze to drizzle over ¼ cup finely chopped fresh basil and additional entire sprigs to adorn the dish

Guidelines

- ❖ The tomato slices should be arranged on a cutting board. After adding ¼ teaspoon of salt and sugar, let it rest for a few minutes so the sugar can dissolve.
- ❖ Place the sliced mozzarella and tomatoes in succession on a serving plate.
- ❖ Evenly distribute the last ¼ teaspoon salt and freshly ground black pepper on top.
- ❖ Pour one tablespoon of olive oil and then the same amount of balsamic glaze on top (you can just eyeball it).
- ❖ Distribute the coarsely chopped basil over top. If desired, garnish the plate with fresh basil sprigs.

Facts about Nutrition

264 calories

19 g of fat

10 g of saturated fat

5 g of carbohydrates

4 g of sugar

Protein: 17 g; Fiber: 1 g

Sodium: 672 milligrams

60 mg of cholesterol

9. Lentil and Sweet Potato Curry

Ingredients

- ❖ For an oil-free dish, use 2 tablespoons of olive oil for soy sauce.
- ❖ One sliced red onion
- ❖ Three minced garlic cloves
- ❖ One large (or two small) sweet potato
- ❖ diced ½ cup red lentils
- ❖ ½ cup vegetable broth

- ❖ One tsp yellow curry powder

- ❖ Half a teaspoon of powdered coriander

- ❖ A smidgeon of cumin powder

- ❖ 1/4 teaspoon powdered garam masala

- ❖ One 15-ounce can of chopped tomatoes

- ❖ One canned (15 oz) creamy coconut milk

Guidelines

- ❖ In a big saucepan, warm up some olive oil over medium heat.

- ❖ Fry the garlic and onion until they become transparent.

- ❖ Meanwhile, thoroughly wash the lentils (a sieve works best for this).

- ❖ Add the chopped tomatoes, lentils, sweet potato cubes, spices, and a little teaspoon of salt.

- ❖ After bringing to a boil, lower the heat, and simmer for ten to twelve minutes covered.

- ❖ After that, pour in the coconut milk and simmer, uncovered, for a further ten minutes. At that point, you might perhaps add some more veggies, such as kale, baby spinach leaves, or olives.

❖ Taste and adjust the seasoning.

❖ Serve with your preferred side dish (rice, naan, etc.) and a squeeze of fresh lime juice.

❖ I also suggest topping with some finely chopped cashews.

❖ It is best enjoyed immediately, but it keeps well in an airtight container and tastes even better the second day!

❖ It is also suitable for freezing!

Dinner

1. Mediterranean Chickpea Stew

Twenty minutes for preparation

Cooking Duration: 30 minutes

50 minutes in total

Yield: 4 servings; Servings: 4.

Ingredients

- ❖ 1/4 cup extra virgin olive oil
- ❖ 2 cups cooked, sodium-free chickpeas, drained
- ❖ 1 cup cherry tomatoes; halved ½ cup vegetable broth
- ❖ 1 big red onion, chopped
- ❖ 1 small bunch Italian parsley; minced
- ❖ 2 cloves garlic; minced
- ❖ 1 small carrot; roughly shredded;
- ❖ 1 small eggplant; cubed;
- ❖ 1 tablespoon of oregano, dry
- ❖ A single tsp of dried thyme

* To taste, add ½ teaspoon of cayenne pepper, salt, and ground black pepper.

Guidelines

* In a Dutch oven over medium heat, warm the olive oil.

* Cook the onion for approximately five minutes, or until it is tender and transparent, in the heated oil. Stir add garlic and parsley and simmer for two minutes.

* Add carrot shreds and stir often for one to two minutes. Add eggplant cubes and cook for two to three minutes.

* Step 2: Add tomatoes and chickpeas. Add the cayenne pepper, thyme, oregano, and broth. Combine and heat through.

* After the veggies are tender and the stew has thickened, reduce the heat and simmer for 15 minutes. If extra broth is needed, add it. Add pepper and salt for seasoning.

Facts about Nutrition (per serving)

326 Calories, 37g Carbs, 10g Protein, and 17g Fat

2. Roasted vegetable and chickpea salad

Serves two to three

15 minutes for preparation

Cook for 20 to 30 minutes.

Ingredients

- One little red onion, sliced into eight equal slices
- Slicing two courgettes thickly
- Cut eight baby sweetcorns in half lengthwise.
- One little red pepper, peeled and sliced into pieces
- Two tsp olive oil
- Eight young cherry or plum tomatoes
- One teaspoon of each of the ground coriander and cumin
- To taste, use half a teaspoon of spicy chili powder.
- one smashed garlic clove
- Six tablespoons of passata or tomato juice
- one and a half tsp balsamic
- freshly ground peppercorns, according to taste
- Rinsed and drained 150g (5 1/2 oz) can of chickpeas (weight drained)

❖ 1-2 teaspoons of freshly chopped basil

Guidelines

❖ Turn the oven on to 220°C, fan 200°C, or gas mark 7. Put the red onion, courgettes, sweetcorn, and red pepper in a roasting tray that is nonstick; pour in one tablespoon of oil and combine well.

❖ Roast for fifteen to twenty minutes. Mix veggies and sprinkle tomatoes on top. Transfer the veggies to a bowl after roasting for a further 5 to 10 minutes, or until they are beginning to turn brown.

❖ Heat the remaining oil in a little skillet. Stir the garlic and spices for one to two minutes. Take the pan off of the burner and mix in the vinegar, black pepper, and tomato juice.

❖ Mix the chickpeas, tomato dressing, and basil with the veggies. Serve warm or cold.

Per 100g, MED salt, low saturated fat
minimal sugar

Energy (kcal) per serving

Percentage of GDA: 211, 11%

Fat: 10g (14%).

1.3g, or 7%, of saturated fat

1.9g, or 32%, of salt

10.7g or 12% sugar

3. Zucchini Noodles with Pesto

Ingredients (Produces 1 Serving)

- ❖ Two medium-sized (around 500g/1 pound) zucchini
- ❖ 1 cup (25g) packed basil leaves - 1/8 cup (15g) pine nuts
- ❖ 45g, or 1/2 cup Parmigiano-Reggiano, grated
- ❖ One clove of garlic
- ❖ Three tablespoons (45 milliliters) of 430 additional virgin olive oil - taste-tested salt

Guidelines

- ❖ Place the zucchini pasta in a strainer, season with salt, and toss to coat. This is how you cook zucchini pasta without using an oven.

- ❖ After 30 minutes, wait, then carefully squeeze out the water and blot thoroughly dry using paper towels.

- ❖ Add 1 tablespoon of olive oil and sauté over medium-high heat for 3 to 5 minutes.

- ❖ There are various varieties of basil available, but Thai basil is less expensive. In my opinion, sweet basil remains the greatest choice for preparing pesto.

- ❖ Always start with the sauce as, once cooked, the zucchini noodles will begin to release water. Serve the noodles immediately after tossing them in the sauce.

- ❖ I increased the salt content of my pesto to avoid adding the last bit of spice just before serving (again since adding salt would extract water from the zucchini, resulting in mushy noodles and watery, thinned-out pesto).

4. Risotto with Butternut Squash

Twenty minutes for preparation

35 minutes for cooking

55 minutes in total

4 servings

Ingredients

- ❖ Two cups of Cubed butternut squash
- ❖ Two teaspoons of butter
- ❖ ½ chopped onion
- ❖ ⅓ cup dry white wine and one cup Arborio rice
- ❖ Five cups of heated chicken broth
- ❖ To taste, add ¼ cup grated Parmesan cheese, salt, and ground black pepper.

Guidelines

- ❖ Squash should be placed in a steamer basket in a saucepan and the basket should be partially submerged in water. Bring the squash to a boil, cover, and steam for 10 to 15 minutes, or until it is soft. Once drained, mash the squash with a fork in a bowl.

- ❖ In a saucepan over medium-high heat, melt the butter. Stir in the rice after cooking and stirring the onion for two minutes, or until it starts to soften. Cook and stir for a further five minutes or so, or until the rice is shiny and the onion is starting to brown on the edges.

- ❖ Add the white wine and stir continuously until it evaporates. Reduce heat to medium and stir in 1/3 of the heated chicken stock and mashed squash.

- ❖ For five to seven minutes, or until the rice has absorbed the chicken broth, cook and stir. Stir in half of the leftover chicken stock and cook, stirring, until the liquid is absorbed. When the risotto is creamy, add the remaining stock and stir once more.

- ❖ Add the Parmesan cheese and season with the pepper and salt.

Facts about Nutrition (per serving)

343 Calories

57g Carbs, 8g Fat, and 7g Protein

5. Tacos with cauliflower and chickpeas

Twenty minutes for preparation

Cooking Time: 25 minutes

45 minutes in total

6 servings; 6 tacos in total.

Ingredients

- ❖ 1 tsp olive oil
- ❖ One tablespoon of lime juice
- ❖ One tsp of chili powder
- ❖ One teaspoon of cumin powder
- ❖ 1/2 teaspoon powdered garlic and 1 teaspoon sea salt
- ❖ One fifteen-ounce can of drained chickpeas
- ❖ One small head of cauliflower, sliced into little pieces

Sauce:

- ❖ One cup of sour cream
- ❖ ¼ cup of freshly chopped cilantro
- ❖ One-third cup of lime juice
- ❖ One tablespoon, to taste, of Sriracha salt
- ❖ Six corn tortillas (6 inches)

Guidelines

* ❖ Set an air fryer to 370 degrees Fahrenheit, or 190 degrees Celsius.
* ❖ In a large bowl, whisk together olive oil, lime juice, cumin, chili powder, salt, and garlic powder. Stir the cauliflower and chickpeas until they are well covered.
* ❖ In a bowl, mix sour cream, lime juice, cilantro, and Sriracha until well blended. Add salt to taste and season.
* ❖ Put the cauliflower mixture into the air fryer's basket. Simmer for 10 minutes, then for a further 10 minutes while stirring.
* ❖ Cook for a further five minutes or to the desired crispness, stirring again.
* ❖ Fill corn tortillas with cauliflower mixture, then cover with sauce.

Facts about Nutrition (per serving)

232 Calories, 28g Carbs, 6g Protein, and 12g Fat

6. Portobello Mushrooms Stuffed

15 minutes for preparation

Cooking Time: 25 minutes

40 minutes in total

Yield: 4 stuffed mushrooms; Servings: 4.

Ingredients

- ❖ Four huge portobello mushroom caps with the gills and stems cut off
- ❖ One spoonful of Italian salad dressing with reduced fat
- ❖ One big egg
- ❖ One garlic clove, chopped salt, and freshly ground black pepper, to taste
- ❖ One 10-oz bag of freshly chopped spinach and ¼ cup of chopped red pepper
- ❖ Grated Parmesan cheese, ¼ cup
- ❖ Partition ¼ cup of shredded mozzarella cheese and ¼ cup of seasoned bread crumbs.

Guidelines

- ❖ Set the oven temperature to 175 degrees Celsius, or 350 degrees Fahrenheit.

- ❖ Apply Italian dressing to the portobello mushrooms on both sides. Place the gill sides of the mushrooms on a baking sheet.

- ❖ Bake for approximately 12 minutes, or until soft, in a preheated oven. Remove any collected juice from the mushrooms.

- ❖ In a large bowl, beat together egg, garlic, salt, and black pepper.

- ❖ Eggs should be well combined with spinach, diced red pepper, Parmesan cheese, three tablespoons of mozzarella cheese, and three teaspoons of bread crumbs.

- ❖ Distribute the spinach mixture among mushroom caps; scatter the remaining 1 tablespoon of mozzarella cheese and 1 tablespoon of bread crumbs over the mushrooms.

- ❖ Put the mushrooms back in the oven and bake for an additional 10 minutes or so, or until the cheese has melted and the topping is golden brown.

Facts about Nutrition (per serving)

161 Calories

10g Protein, 11g Carbs, and 9g Fat

7. spinach and mushroom lasagna

Servings: 6-8

Twenty-five minutes for preparation

Two hours in total

Ingredients for pasta cooked from scratch

Semolina flour (two cups + more for dusting)

Ingredients for filling:

- ❖ Olive oil, six teaspoons
- ❖ 3 minced garlic cloves
- ❖ Three little yellow onions, cut thinly, with kosher salt

* Three pounds (or 1361 grams) of thinly sliced cremini mushrooms
* thirty ounces (or 850 grams) of defrosted, well-drained, and coarsely chopped frozen spinach
* Six cups of mozzarella shredded
* Three cups of freshly ground black pepper and ricotta cheese, to taste

Ingredients for bechamel:

* Four tsp unsalted butter
* ⅓ cup flour for all purposes
* 4 glasses (946 ml) of whole milk
* To taste, add kosher salt
* Freshly ground black pepper.

Ingredients for lasagna:

* One pound (454 grams) of fresh pasta
* Four tsp olive oil
* Grate 1/4 cup of parmesan cheese recently.

Guidelines

❖ To make the pasta, use a mixer equipped with a dough hook to combine the flour with ⅔ cup|158 ml water. Add more water as required to make the mixture smooth and somewhat stretchy.

❖ Refrigerate the dough for at least two hours after wrapping it in plastic wrap. Pasta dough may be stored for up to three months or refrigerated for up to five days.

❖ Cut the dough into four pieces and use them to construct the pasta. Dust a work surface with flour. Working with a single piece of dough at a time, cover the remaining dough with a moist cloth. Place the portion on a work surface after running it through the pasta maker's second-thinnest setting. Continue doing this with the remaining dough pieces.

❖ Prepare the filling: In a large saucepan, heat the oil over medium-high heat. Season with salt and add the onions and garlic. Simmer for 4 minutes, or until tender. Cook for a further eight minutes or until the mushrooms are tender.

❖ After the mushroom mixture has cooled down enough to handle, transfer it to a colander and let it drain for

20 minutes. Finally, push out any liquid that remains. After transferring the mushrooms to a large bowl, mix in the spinach, ricotta, and three cups of mozzarella. Season with salt and pepper.

❖ Prepare the bechamel: In a 6-quart saucepan, melt the butter over medium-high heat. Add the flour, then boil for two minutes.

❖ Add the milk and simmer for 8 to 10 minutes, stirring often, until thickened. Add salt and pepper for seasoning, then stir in the mushroom mixture.

❖ Put the lasagna together: If you're using store-bought pasta, start by boiling a big pot of well-salted water. After adding the lasagna sheets, cook for ten minutes or until it's al dente. After draining, gently stir with two tablespoons of olive oil.

❖ If you're using our handmade pasta, divide the dough into four equal portions, covering the remaining portions with a towel while you work with each one. Shape the portion into a about 3-by-4-inch rectangle and run it through your pasta maker's biggest roller setting.

❖ After folding the dough into a rectangle, proceed again, narrowing the setting after each pass, until the dough passes through the second-thinnest setting.

❖ Continue with the remaining dough pieces until you have four spaghetti sheets that are two to three feet long and five inches broad. After applying a semolina dusting, cut each sheet into 13-inch lengths. Avoid boiling.

❖ Set oven temperature to 375°F. Fill a 9 by 13-inch baking dish with the remaining 2 teaspoons of oil. Line the dish with three lasagna sheets if you're using store-bought noodles. Place two sheets of handmade pasta in the dish.

❖ Evenly distribute 2 cups of filling over the pasta, then top with ½ cup of the leftover mozzarella. Put three more spaghetti sheets on top, then keep adding layers of mozzarella and filling. When you reach the last layer, sprinkle the remaining filling, one cup of mozzarella, and Parmesan cheese on top.

❖ After baking for 35 to 40 minutes, lightly cover with aluminum foil. After removing the foil, preheat the oven to broil. After baking for a further five minutes, take the lasagna out of the oven. Before serving, let it settle for five to ten minutes.

8. Primavera Spaghetti Squash

15 minutes for preparation

Cooking Duration: 30 minutes

45 minutes in total

Six servings

Ingredients

- ❖ 1 spaghetti squash
- ❖ Two teaspoons of pure olive oil
- ❖ one sliced onion
- ❖ one big minced garlic clove
- ❖ One big zucchini, sliced into small pieces
- ❖ One sliced green bell pepper
- ❖ One tablespoon of freshly ground black pepper
- ❖ Dried Italian herb spice, to taste
- ❖ 1/2 cup finely sliced tomato
- ❖ 1/4 cup of feta cheese, crumbled

- ❖ Using a fork, pierce the spaghetti squash shell and transfer it to a plate that is safe to use in the microwave. Cook on high for 12 minutes. Wait till it's safe to handle.

- ❖ Halve the squash lengthwise, then scrape out the seeds. Pull the meat from the shell with a fork and transfer it to a large dish, fluffing the meat to break up the threads as much as possible.

- ❖ In a big skillet over medium heat, warm up the olive oil. In heated oil, cook and stir onion for approximately 3 minutes, or until it is just soft. Cook and stir the garlic for a further three minutes. Add zucchini and green bell pepper to the mixture; add black pepper and Italian herb spice.

- ❖ Transfer the tomatoes to the skillet. After 3 to 5 minutes, or until the tomatoes are barely warmed through, continue cooking. Squash strands should be added to the skillet and stirred evenly. To serve, add feta cheese and mix once more.

Facts about Nutrition (per serving)

158 Calories

5g Protein, 16g Carbs, and 10g Fat

9. Chickpea and Sweet Potato Vegan Curry

Ten minutes for preparation

Cooking Time: 20 minutes

30 minutes in total

Six servings

Ingredients

- Three teaspoons of extra virgin olive oil
- One sliced onion and two minced garlic cloves
- two tsp finely chopped, fresh ginger root
- One fifteen-ounce can of drained chickpeas
- One 14.5-oz can of chopped tomatoes
- One 14-oz can of coconut milk
- One diced sweet potato and one tablespoon of garam masala
- One teaspoon of cumin powder
- One tsp ground turmeric, one tsp salt, and one tsp red chili flakes
- One cup of baby spinach

Guidelines

- ❖ Heat the oil in a skillet over medium heat.
- ❖ In heated oil, cook onion, garlic, and ginger for approximately five minutes, or until softened.
- ❖ Add the sweet potato, tomatoes, coconut milk, and chickpeas. After bringing to a boil, lower the heat, and simmer for 15 minutes or until the food is soft.
- ❖ Add garam masala, cumin, turmeric, salt, and chili flakes for seasoning. Just before serving, add the spinach.

Facts about Nutrition (per serving)

293 Calories, 5g Protein, 22g Carbs, and 22g Fat

11. Mushroom and Lentil Shepherd's Pie

Ingredients

- ❖ lentils
- ❖ Sweet potatoes
- ❖ Paste made with tomatoes
- ❖ Soy sauce
- ❖ The onion

- ❖ Nooch Cornstarch

- ❖ fungi

- ❖ frozen vegetables

- ❖ Garlic

- ❖ dehydrated herbs

- ❖ Vegan milk with veggie broth

Guidelines

- ❖ Don't overcook the lentils; simply simmer them until they're soft. I suggest combining one cup of dry lentils with three cups of water and simmering them together (or following the packet directions). They will be ready when you need them since they cook rapidly.

- ❖ Incorporate the soy sauce, tomato paste, and cornstarch into the vegetable broth as well. Mix well until no clumps remain.

- ❖ Quarter and peel the potatoes. Move them to a medium-sized saucepan and add water to cover. After bringing to a boil, reduce the heat to low-medium and simmer the potatoes for 20 minutes or until they are tender.

❖ After draining, put the potatoes back in the saucepan. Return the saucepan to the burner and let them dry out for one or two minutes (the water will evaporate). Next, mash the potatoes as smooth as possible using a hand masher.

❖ Once you've added some salt and vegan milk, mash the nutritional yeast and continue adding milk until you get the required consistency. For perfectly fluffy potatoes, I also like using an electric beater to combine the mixture at the end.

❖ On medium heat, brown onions in a big skillet, turning often, for approximately 5 minutes. Apply a little amount of oil or water.

❖ Cook for a further five minutes after adding the dry herbs, garlic, and mushrooms. Stir in the frozen veggies after that. Simmer for a further five minutes, or until they are thawed. After the vegetables are done, add the broth mixture to the pan along with the cooked and drained lentils. Once again, stir regularly and return to a low simmer. Once simmered, it should thicken fast. Take off the heat source. Taste and adjust the seasoning.

- ❖ Thaw the whole bag of frozen corn by either microwaving it for a short while or soaking it in hot water for a few minutes.

- ❖ After thoroughly draining, add a generous amount of salt and 1 ½ cups of the corn to a blender along with the vegan milk.

- ❖ Blend until fairly smooth—perfectionism is not necessary—then return to the remaining whole kernels—roughly 1 to 1 ½ cups—and stir..

- ❖ Transfer the lentil mixture to a big square or rectangular baking dish and use a large spoon to level it evenly. Next, distribute the creamed corn evenly with a spoon after scattering it over.

- ❖ Mashed potatoes should be added last, strewn on top, and the surface should be smoothed. To help brown and crisp the top layer of the potatoes, use a fork to put some texture on them.

- ❖ Bake for approximately 25 to 30 minutes, or until the top is golden brown and the edges are bubbling.

- ❖ Finally, broil for a few minutes while keeping a close eye on everything! Before consuming, let the shepherd's pie rest for five to ten minutes.

❖ Up close, a fork is taking a piece out of a vegan shepherd's pie with lentils and mushrooms.

Cooking Advice

If you want to prevent a gummy texture in your mashed potatoes, don't combine them.

If you want the lentils to have a richer taste, feel free to add some red wine. Once done, add roughly ½ cup to the pan of vegetables. Next, add the broth mixture after letting the wine reduce.

12. Stuffed bell pepper with quinoa and black beans

Ingredients

❖ Bell peppers: You may use any color of pepper, but because of their sweet taste, I like red or orange. Green works too, however, roasted it might sometimes taste harsh.

❖ Black beans: Use cooked dry beans or drain and rinse canned beans before using. Select beans labeled "no salt added" for a better choice.

- ❖ Diced tomatoes with a kick: For a little additional oomph, try fire-roasted tomatoes or just plain diced tomatoes.

- ❖ Quinoa provides additional nutrition and a nutty taste. Quinoa of any hue works well. Rinse the quinoa before cooking, if possible.

- ❖ Corn: tinned, frozen, or fresh. Fire-roasted corn is really good if you can get it.

- ❖ Seasoning for tacos: This includes cumin, chili powder, onion powder, and garlic powder. You are welcome to prepare your taco seasoning or just purchase a package.

Guidelines

- ❖ First, get the quinoa filling ready. Add dry quinoa, garlic cloves, and optional jalapeño (if you enjoy spicy food) after sautéing onion in olive oil until it becomes soft.

- ❖ To bring out the natural taste of this grain, toast the quinoa for one minute. Add fluids and spices and stir.

❖ Over high heat, bring the quinoa to a boil. Lower the heat to a simmer while covering. Simmer for 15 minutes or until the quinoa is cooked and fluffy.

❖ Mix in the drained tomatoes, frozen corn (no need to defrost), black beans, and ½ cup of shredded cheese.

❖ Put the peppers together in a cast iron or lightly greased baking dish. Fill each pepper with a cup of the black bean and quinoa mixture. Using a spoon, press down on the quinoa mixture to ensure that it is packed securely. Add cheese shreds on top of the peppers.

❖ Bake for 30 minutes while covered with foil. After ten minutes, take off the foil and continue baking the cheese until it becomes brown and bubbling.

SNACKS

1. Hummus and Veggie Sticks

Ingredients

- ❖ One cup of kabuli chana, or chickpeas
- ❖ Two tablespoons powdered sesame seeds
- ❖ Two tablespoons of lemon juice
- ❖ two to three cloves of garlic
- ❖ One tablespoon of sesame or olive oil
- ❖ half a teaspoon of jeera powder, or cumin powder
- ❖ A tsp of chili powder
- ❖ according to taste, pink salt

Instructions

- ❖ First, give chickpeas a 6 to 7 hour soak.
- ❖ Soak the chickpeas and add enough water to the pressure cooker (five to six whistles).
- ❖ Second, place the toasted sesame seeds in a mixer grinder and grind them finely to a powder.

- ❖ And finally. Add the curd, sesame powder, and chickpeas to another jar in your mixer. rock salt and minced garlic. the powdered jeera and oil. Mix everything to create a smooth paste. Press a lemon. If necessary, add more water to fully mix everything.

- ❖ Now place the hummus in a dish for serving. Add a little oil and season with chili powder. Add coriander leaves as a garnish.

- ❖ Cut the bell pepper, cucumber, carrots, and celery into sticks and place them in a different dish. Accompany hummus with vegetable sticks.

- ❖ Along with falafel, you may also enjoy hummus dip.

- ❖ Pita chips go very well with hummus.

- ❖ Spread it on your sandwiches as a nutritious alternative.

- ❖ Pour some as a creamy dressing over your salad.

- ❖ Simply eat a tablespoon of hummus as you would peanut butter.

- ❖ Keep it in a sealed container. It should keep well in the refrigerator for four to five days.

2. Roasted Chickpeas

Five minutes for preparation

Cooking Period: 40 minutes

45 minutes in total

4 servings

Ingredients

- ❖ 1 (15-oz) bag of drained chickpeas (garbanzo beans)
- ❖ Two tsp olive oil
- ❖ One garlic salt pinch, or to taste
- ❖ One cayenne pepper sprinkle, or to taste.
- ❖ one salt pinch, or to taste

Guidelines

- ❖ Heat the oven to 450 degrees Fahrenheit, or 230 degrees Celsius.
- ❖ To dry the chickpeas, blot them with a paper towel.
- ❖ Olive oil and chickpeas should be combined in a dish.
- ❖ Toss again and season with salt, cayenne, and garlic salt to taste.
- ❖ Arrange the chickpeas on a baking sheet with a rim.

❖ Roast for 30 to 40 minutes in a preheated oven, or until browned and crispy; keep an eye on them to prevent burning.

Facts about Nutrition (per serving)

161 Calories, 19g Carbs, 4g Protein, and 8g Fat

3. Greek Yogurt and Berry Parfait

There are two servings.

Five minutes for preparation

One minute for cooking

187 kcal of calories

Ingredients

❖ One cup of fat-free Greek yogurt

❖ 2 TSP vanilla protein powder (Orgain was our option).

❖ One teaspoon of pure vanilla essence

❖ Six ounces of raspberries

❖ Six ounces of blackberries

❖ Six ounces of strawberries

Guidelines

- ❖ Strawberries, blackberries, and raspberries should all be cleaned and dried. Slice the strawberries into more manageable chunks.
- ❖ The vanilla protein powder, extract, and fat-free Greek yogurt should all be combined in a dish.
- ❖ Put each parfait together in a jar. After each layer of fruit, divide the yogurt mixture among the jars. To keep the berries fresh, enjoy them soon after preparing them.

4. Roasted Edamame with Sea Salt and Pepper

Ingredients:

- ❖ One dozen twelve-ounce shelled edamame (fresh or frozen and defrosted)
- ❖ 1/4 tsp sea salt, or according to your taste
- ❖ Add pepper to taste, ground
- ❖ Cooking Mist

Guidelines:

* ❖ Preheat the oven to 425 degrees.
* ❖ Apply cooking spray to a baking sheet. If the edamame is damp from defrosting, pat them dry.
* ❖ Arrange the edamame pieces on the sheet pan.
* ❖ Apply baking spray on the edamame and season with salt & pepper.
* ❖ Bake them for thirty to thirty-five minutes, or until they are crisp and golden brown. as they're preparing food. Every ten minutes, shake the pan to ensure equal browning.
* ❖ Allow to cool and proceed to serve.

5. Cucumber and Avocado Salsa

Ten minutes to prepare.

Cooking Period: Minutes

Time to Chill: 20 Minutes

30 minutes in total

There are four servings.

Ingredients

- ❖ Two ripe, diced avocados
- ❖ Two tsp freshly squeezed lemon juice from ½ lemon
- ❖ One chopped and cleaned English cucumber
- ❖ Diced red onion (two tablespoons) and ¼ cup fresh dill
- ❖ One spoonful of sugar
- ❖ 1/4 cup olive oil
- ❖ 1 ½ teaspoons red wine vinegar
- ❖ Salt and pepper to taste

Guidelines

- ❖ In a medium bowl, gently combine avocado and lemon juice.
- ❖ Combine all remaining ingredients by giving them a little shake.
- ❖ Let it cool for twenty minutes before serving.

6. Cheese and Whole-Grain Crackers

1.15 hours for preparation

Cooking Period: 15 minutes

1 hour and 30 minutes in total

Ingredients

- ❖ Eight-ounce block of strong cheddar cheese
- ❖ Four tablespoons (half a stick) of cold, unsalted butter
- ❖ One cup of whole-grain flour (or any other kind of flour)
- ❖ Half a spoonful of lukewarm water

Guidelines

- ❖ Start the oven at 375 degrees Fahrenheit.
- ❖ Shred a block of cheese using a shredder or food processor attachment.
- ❖ Cut the butter stick in half into 1-inch chunks.
- ❖ Put the flour, butter, and cheese into the food processor and pulse until the mixture resembles pebbles.

* Water should be added one spoonful at a time, and pulverized until dough forms. If needed, add one additional tablespoon of water.
* Refrigerate the dough for one hour after wrapping it in plastic wrap.
* Pat dough to a thickness of 1/8 inch, then cut into 1x1 inch squares. Perhaps puncture a hole in the center (optional).
* Place on parchment paper or a silicone mat, and bake for 12 to 15 minutes at 375 degrees F.
* After 5 to 10 minutes of sitting, keep in an airtight container.

Remark

To change the taste, use a different variety of cheese!

Facts about Nutrition (per serving)

121 calories

9 g of fat

6 g of carbohydrates

4 g of protein

7. Vegetable Spring Rolls

Twenty minutes for preparation

15 minutes is the cooking time.

Thirty-five minutes total

Six servings

Ingredients (240 ML = US CUP)

For the Filling

- Three cups of shredded cabbage
- Shredded one medium carrot, approximately ½ cup
- 1/4 cup finely chopped bell pepper or capsicum
- Two distinct spring onion sprigs (white and green)
- one or two tsp oil
- One or two tsp soy sauce
- ¼ to ½ teaspoons of black pepper powder and 1 teaspoon of rice vinegar
- salt, if necessary
- Half a noodle cake or one cup of cooked noodles (optional)

Ingredients for or Vegetable Spring Rolls

- ❖ Six frozen spring roll wrappers
- ❖ One tablespoon of oil for baking or one cup for deep-frying

Guidelines

- ❖ Heat some oil in a skillet and sauté the whites of spring onions.
- ❖ Add every vegetable, except the onion greens.
- ❖ Fry over high heat until crisp but not fully cooked.
- ❖ Add vinegar and soy sauce. Blend well.
- ❖ Add the onion greens, a little bit of salt, and pepper. Stir and turn off the heat.
- ❖ Boil noodles al dente if you want to use them. After thorough rinsing, drain entirely. Stir-fry them for a minute after adding them to the vegetables.
- ❖ Add one teaspoon more soy sauce. Add a little pepper and salt.
- ❖ Allow this to cool fully.

Guidelines for Spring Rolls

* For five to seven minutes, cover the frozen sheets with a moist towel or as directed on the package.

* After spreading out one wrapper, add a dollop of filling.

* Roll one edge in the direction of the stuffing's inner side.

* Transfer the sides to the middle. To seal, moisten the leftover edge of the wrapper and roll it.

* Without a covering, they will get dry.

* Heat the oil to a sufficient temperature. Drop a little piece of wrapper into the oil to be sure.

* It rises in the oil without browning if the temperature is high enough.

* When the oil is heated, add the rolls and stir-fry them evenly until brown. Take them off with kitchen paper.

* Serve hot spring rolls with ketchup on the side.

Guidelines for vegetable Spring Roll

* Take at least fifteen minutes to preheat the oven to 220 C.

* Give the spring rolls a thorough oil brushing.

* After sprinkling a little oil on a baking pan, bake for 12 to 13 minutes.
* A wired rack is also functional. After six more minutes of baking, turn them if necessary.
* Serve warm spring rolls with any kind of sauce.

8. Trail Mix with Nuts and Dried Fruits

30 minutes in total

Make 1 3⁄4 cups (7 servings) in the yield.

Ingredients

* Half a cup of uncooked almonds
* 1/4 cup uncooked cashews
* ½ cup uncooked walnut halves
* Kosher salt or sea salt?
* Half a cup of golden raisins
* ¼ cup of cranberries dried
* 1/4 cup of dried apricots
* Half a cup of banana chips

Guidelines

* ❖ Set oven temperature to 350°. Spread the nuts out on a baking sheet after tossing them with a little salt.
* ❖ Toast for ten minutes, stirring halfway through, until golden.
* ❖ Allow the nuts to cool fully. Combine the dried fruits and nuts.

9. Avocado and Tomato salad

15 minutes for preparation

15 minutes in total

Yield: 4 servings; Servings: 4.

Ingredients

* ❖ ¼ cup extra virgin olive oil, ½ cup balsamic vinegar, and 1 teaspoon Dijon mustard.
* ❖ One dash of freshly ground black pepper
* ❖ One avocado, cut, pitted, and peeled
* ❖ Two little tomatoes, each divided into eight wedges

- ❖ Mix the mustard, olive oil, balsamic vinegar, and pepper in a small bowl.
- ❖ Arrange the tomato and avocado slices on one large serving dish, or separate plates, in the pattern of a wheel's spokes.
- ❖ Serve right away after gently drizzling with the dressing.

Facts about Nutrition (per serving)

236 energy

11g Carbs, 22g Fat, and 2g Protein

10. Cottage Cheese and Pineapple Bowl

Ingredients

250 grams of cottage cheese

One spoonful of honey

One pineapple

Guidelines

❖ To make this breakfast meal, first coarsely crumble the cottage cheese into a bowl.

❖ Now, chop the pineapple into the appropriate size and shape on a cutting board, then add it to the bowl along with the crumbled cottage cheese.

❖ After that, thoroughly mix in the honey in the dish of cottage cheese.

❖ Make sure to drizzle honey over the cottage cheese and pineapple.

❖ Enjoy it right away served with a glass of fresh juice!

Dessert

1. Chocolate Avocado Mousse (pudding)

Ten minutes for preparation

Extra Time: thirty minutes

40 minutes in total

4 servings

Ingredients

- ❖ Two big avocados that have been diced, pitted, and peeled
- ❖ ½ cup chocolate powder, unsweetened
- ❖ Half a cup of brown sugar
- ❖ One-third cup of coconut milk
- ❖ two tsp of essence from vanilla
- ❖ One pinch of ground cinnamon

Guidelines

- ❖ Smoothly combine avocados, brown sugar, cocoa powder, coconut milk, vanilla, and cinnamon in a blender.
- ❖ The pudding should be transferred to a lidded container and refrigerated for about half an hour.

Facts about Nutrition (per serving)

400 Calories, 46g Carbs, 5g Protein, and 26g Fat

2. Baked Apple with Cinnamon

15 minutes for preparation

15 minutes for cooking

30 minutes in total

4 servings

Ingredients

- ❖ Four apples, like Honeycrisp or Granny Smith
- ❖ Half a cup of brown sugar
- ❖ four tsp of butter

❖ two tsp finely ground cinnamon

Guidelines

- ❖ Compile every component.
- ❖ Set the oven temperature to 175 degrees Celsius, or 350 degrees Fahrenheit.
- ❖ Take off the core, leaving a well on the top of each apple.
- ❖ Put one spoonful of butter and two teaspoons of brown sugar into each apple. Transfer to a baking dish that is not too deep and top with cinnamon.
- ❖ Bake in the preheated oven for 15 to 30 minutes, depending on the size of the apples, or until the sugar starts to caramelize and the apples are soft.

Facts about Nutrition (per serving)

270 Calories

45g Carbs /12g Fat

One gram of protein

3. Chia Seed Pudding with Berries

Ingredients

- One cup of almond milk
- Two tsp honey
- One-fourth cup of chia seeds
- One cup of strawberries
- Half a teaspoon of extract from vanilla

Guidelines

- Puree the strawberries.
- Put the strawberries and almond milk into a blender jar. After blending until a homogeneous paste is achieved, pour the mixture into a serving dish.
- Include the chia seeds.
- Mix the vanilla essence, honey, and chia seeds into the strawberry mixture. Blend the items well using a spoon.
- Chill and savor!

❖ To allow the pudding to set, put the bowl in the fridge for a bit. After it has set, top with some fresh strawberries and serve cold.

Advice

You may also add flaxseeds, almonds, and berry jam to make it even more delicious. You may enhance the flavor by adding dates.

4. Frozen Banana Bites

Thirty minutes for preparation

1 hour 45 minutes for cooking

2 hours and 15 minutes in total

Yield: 48 servings; Servings: 48

Ingredients

❖ One cup of peanut butter

❖ Four bananas, cut into rounds of one inch

❖ Eight one-ounce semisweet chocolate squares

❖ One tablespoon of shortening

❖ ⅓ cup baking bits with toffee

- Put the waxed paper on a baking pan.

- Place a little amount of peanut butter on top of every slice of banana. Take a toothpick and poke it through the banana's peanut butter coating. Put the banana bits on the baking sheet that has been prepared, and freeze for 30 to 60 minutes.

- In a double boiler set over boiling water, melt the shortening and chocolate, stirring often and scraping down the sides with a rubber spatula to prevent burning.

- Put parchment paper on the second baking sheet.

- Take out two to four bits of banana at a time from the freezer, and then cover each mouthful with chocolate mixture.

- Scatter toffee pieces over each covered banana bite before placing them on the second baking sheet. Continue until all of the bites have a coating.

- Put the banana bits back in the freezer for at least an hour to solidify. Before serving, let the bites remain at room temperature for about fifteen minutes.

Facts about Nutrition (per serving)

76 Calories, 2g Protein, 7g Carbs, and 5g Fat

5. Blueberry Sorbet

20 minutes in total

10 minutes in preparation

100 calories

4 serving

Ingredients

- ❖ Two cups of blueberries, frozen
- ❖ 1 sprinkle kosher salt,
- ❖ 1/2 tablespoon honey,
- ❖ 1/4 teaspoon lime zest, and waffle cone as needed
- ❖ Two tablespoons of sugar

Guidelines

- ❖ Combine honey with blueberries.

- ❖ First, place the blueberries in a basin and remove the seeds. This is the dessert recipe. Now, combine the honey, sugar, salt, and lemon zest in the same bowl and well stir.

- ❖ Place the blueberry mixture into the jar of the blender and pulse at high speed. Ensure that the mixture solidifies into a paste.

- ❖ Sift this mixture to get rid of the bigger blueberry fragments. Transfer this mixture into a jar and seal it shut. Put this in the freezer.

- ❖ After it's frozen, remove it, spoon it onto a waffle cone, and serve it right away for consumption!

6. Greek Yogurt Parfait with Dark Chocolate

Ingredients

- ❖ Half a cup of melted dark chocolate, chopped coarsely.

- ❖ one-third cup of heavy cream

- ❖ Half a cup of whipped cream

- ❖ three yolks from eggs

- ❖ two tsp sugar

- ❖ 1/4 cup of coffee, espresso

Guidelines

- ❖ Place the egg yolks in a bowl and whisk in the sugar until the mixture becomes light yellow. Pour in the espresso coffee and the melted dark chocolate. Blend well.

- ❖ Beat the cream in another dish until firm peaks form, then stir it into the chocolate mixture. Add the egg whites to the chocolate mixture after beating them in a separate dish until firm peaks form. Stir well. Transfer the chocolate mousse onto dessert dishes and refrigerate for four hours.

- ❖ Prepare the dark chocolate mousse. Few desserts can match the sophistication, beauty, and delectability of a well-made mousse. Serve the mousse cold and garnish with whipped cream.

7. Almond and Date Energy Balls

22 minutes in total

Preparation Duration: 7 minutes

242 calories

4 servings

Ingredients

- 250 grams of black dates
- One teaspoon of green cardamom powder
- One cup of almonds
- One dash of salt for marination
- two cups of coconut powder

Guidelines

- Fill a pot with two to three cups of water and bring it to a boil. Place the dates in a sieve after pitting them.
- To soften the dates, place this sieve over a pot of boiling water.
- Stir until pulpy in step three. This should take ten to fifteen minutes. Take off the heat and place in a food

processor with the almonds, salt, and cardamom powder.

❖ Pulse the ingredients until they resemble dough.

❖ Transfer to a bowl and cover. Refrigerate for thirty minutes.

❖ Using a tablespoon, divide the mixture equally and form into balls.

❖ Swirl in the coconut powder very gently and leave aside. Savor!

8. Strawberry and Basil Popsicles

Ingredients

❖ 1 pint of fresh, washed, and chopped strawberries

❖ 4 tablespoons of sugar, or less according to how sweet your strawberries are.

❖ 10 dry, clean basil leaves

❖ optional sweetened condensed milk

Guidelines

- ❖ Heat the sugar and strawberries until they become tender.

- ❖ In a blender, puree the strawberries and basil until smooth, then set aside to chill.

- ❖ Using sweetened condensed milk as desired, pour the strawberry-basil mixture into the popsicle molds in alternating cycles.

- ❖ Before serving, freeze the popsicles for four to six hours.

- ❖ Reminder: If the popsicle is difficult to remove from the mold, just give the mold outside a 30-second rinse with room-temperature tap water.

9. Pumpkin pie smoothie

Preparation Time: Five minutes in total
One serving yields one smoothie.

Ingredients

- ❖ One-half cup pureed pumpkin
- ❖ A quarter cup of almond milk
- ❖ (Optional) ½ cup of cold water
- ❖ One tablespoon of pumpkin syrup

- ❖ ½ teaspoon spice for pumpkin pie

- ❖ Two packets of erythritol-stevia sweeteners, or to taste

- ❖ Five ice cubes (optional)

Guidelines

- ❖ In a blender, combine pumpkin puree, almond milk, water, sugar, pumpkin pie spice, and pumpkin syrup.

- ❖ Blend for 5 to 10 seconds, or until thoroughly incorporated. Blend in the ice cubes until smooth.

Facts about Nutrition (per serving)

77 Calories, 17g Carbs, 2g Fat, and 2g Protein

10. Berry and Oat Crumble Bars

15 minutes for preparation

35 minutes for cooking

50 minutes in total

24 servings

24 bars are the yield.

Ingredients

- ❖ 1 ½ cups flour (all-purpose)
- ❖ 1/2 cup instant-cooking oats
- ❖ a half-cup of white sugar, separated
- ❖ One-half teaspoon of ground cinnamon
- ❖ One-half teaspoon of baking soda
- ❖ Half a cup of chilled, diced butter
- ❖ Two cups of blueberries
- ❖ two tsp cornstarch
- ❖ two tsp lemon juice

Guidelines

- ❖ Set the oven's temperature to 375°F, or 190°C. Grease a 9 by 13-inch baking dish.
- ❖ In a large bowl, mix flour, oats, 1 cup sugar, cinnamon, and baking soda. Using two knives or a pastry blender, cut in butter until the mixture resembles coarse crumbs; set aside approximately 2 cups for the topping. Using your fingers, press the remaining oat mixture into the baking dish to create a crust.

❖ In a saucepan, bring the blueberries, remaining 1/2 cup sugar, cornstarch, and lemon juice to a boil. Stir continuously and cook for approximately 2 minutes, or until the mixture thickens. Sprinkle the leftover oat mixture on top after spreading it over the crust.

❖ Bake for approximately 25 minutes in a preheated oven, or until the topping is just beginning to brown. Allow to cool fully before slicing into 24 bars.

Facts about Nutrition (per serving)

157 Calories

24g Carbs, 6g Fat, and 2g Protein

Bonus

A five-week meal plan

Week 1

Monday

Breakfast: Greek Yogurt Parfait

Lunch: Chickpea and Spinach Quesadilla

Dinner: Mushroom and Spinach Lasagna

Snack: Roasted Chickpeas

Tuesday

Breakfast: Quinoa Breakfast Bowl

Lunch: Mediterranean Chickpea Salad

Dinner: Zucchini Noodles with Pesto

Snack: Greek Yogurt and Berry Parfait

Wednesday:

Breakfast: Avocado Toast with Tomato

Lunch: Sweet Potato and Lentil Curry

Dinner: Vegan Sweet Potato Chickpea Curry

Snack: Hummus and Veggie Sticks

Thursday:

Breakfast: Berry and Nut Oatmeal

Lunch: Caprese Salad with Balsamic Glaze

Dinner: Butternut Squash Risotto

Snack: Trail Mix with Nuts and Dried Fruits

Friday:

Breakfast: Sweet Potato and Black Bean Breakfast Burrito

Lunch: Chickpea and Spinach Quesadilla

Dinner: Vegan Sweet Potato Chickpea Curry

Snack: Cucumber and Avocado Salsa

Saturday:

Breakfast: Blueberry Almond Overnight Oats

Lunch: Caprese Salad with Balsamic Glaze

Dinner: Spaghetti Squash Primavera

Snack: Roasted Edamame with Sea Salt and Pepper

Sunday:

Breakfast: Chia Seed Pudding with Mango

Lunch: Sweet Potato and Lentil Curry

Dinner: Mushroom and Lentil Shepherd's Pie

Snack: Cheese and Whole-Grain Crackers

Week 2

Monday:

Breakfast: Greek Yogurt Parfait

Lunch: Vegan Coconut-Lentil Curry with Sweet Potatoes

Dinner: Cauliflower and Chickpea Tacos

Snack: Roasted Chickpeas

Tuesday:

Breakfast: Quinoa Breakfast Bowl

Lunch: Roasted Vegetable and Hummus Wrap

Dinner: Mushroom and Spinach Lasagna

Snack: Greek Yogurt and Berry Parfait

Wednesday:

Breakfast: Avocado Toast with Tomato

Lunch: Cauliflower Fried Rice

Dinner: Zucchini Noodles with Pesto

Snack: Hummus and Veggie Sticks

Thursday:

Breakfast: Berry and Nut Oatmeal

Lunch: Lentil and Vegetable Soup

Dinner: Eggplant and Chickpea Stew (Mediterranean Chickpea Stew)

Snack: Trail Mix with Nuts and Dried Fruits

Friday:

Breakfast: Sweet Potato and Black Bean Breakfast Burrito

Lunch: Chickpea and Spinach Quesadilla

Dinner: Vegan Sweet Potato Chickpea Curry

Snack: Cucumber and Avocado Salsa

Saturday:

Breakfast: Berry and Nut Oatmeal

Lunch: Roasted Vegetable and Hummus Wrap

Dinner: Zucchini Noodles with Pesto

Snack: Avocado and Tomato Salad

Sunday:

Breakfast: Greek Yogurt Parfait

Lunch: Lentil and Vegetable Soup

Dinner: Stuffed Bell Pepper with Quinoa and Black Beans

Snack: Roasted Chickpeas

Week 3

Monday:

Breakfast: Black Bean Breakfast Bowl

Lunch: Chickpea and Spinach Quesadilla

Dinner: Butternut Squash Risotto

Snack: Cheese and Whole-Grain Crackers

Tuesday:

Breakfast: Blueberry Almond Overnight Oats

Lunch: Caprese Salad with Balsamic Glaze

Dinner: Spaghetti Squash Primavera

Snack: Roasted Edamame with Sea Salt and Pepper

Wednesday:

Breakfast: Chia Seed Pudding with Mango

Lunch: Sweet Potato and Lentil Curry

Dinner: Vegan Sweet Potato Chickpea Curry

Snack: Cucumber and Avocado Salsa

Thursday:

Breakfast: Spinach and Feta Omelette

Lunch: Mediterranean Chickpea Salad

Dinner: Stuffed Bell Pepper with Quinoa and Black Beans

Snack: Avocado and Tomato Salad

Friday:

Breakfast: Spinach and Feta Omelette

Lunch: Cauliflower and Chickpea Tacos

Dinner: Eggplant and Chickpea Stew (Mediterranean Chickpea Stew)

Snack: Roasted Chickpeas

Saturday:

Breakfast: Whole Wheat Pancakes

Lunch: Chickpea and Spinach Quesadilla

Dinner: Spaghetti Squash Primavera

Snack: Cheese and Whole-Grain Crackers

Sunday:

Breakfast: Chia Seed Pudding with Berries

Lunch: Lentil and Vegetable Soup

Dinner: Stuffed Portobello Mushrooms

Snack: Greek Yogurt and Berry Parfait

Week 4

Monday:

Breakfast: Whole Wheat Pancakes

Lunch: Roasted Vegetable and Hummus Wrap

Dinner: Spaghetti Squash Primavera

Snack: Trail Mix with Nuts and Dried Fruits

Tuesday:

Breakfast: Chia Seed Pudding with Berries

Lunch: Lentil and Vegetable Soup

Dinner: Stuffed Portobello Mushrooms

Snack: Greek Yogurt and Berry Parfait

Wednesday:

Breakfast: Cottage Cheese and Pineapple Bowl

Lunch: Vegan Sweet Potato Chickpea Curry

Dinner: Cauliflower Fried Rice

Snack: Hummus and Veggie Sticks

Thursday:

Breakfast: Avocado Toast with Tomato

Lunch: Mediterranean Chickpea Salad

Dinner: Cauliflower and Chickpea Tacos

Snack: Roasted Edamame with Sea Salt and Pepper

Friday

Breakfast: Chia Seed Pudding with Berries

Lunch: Lentil and Vegetable Soup

Dinner: Mushroom and Lentil Shepherd's Pie

Snack: Cucumber and Avocado Salsa

Saturday

Breakfast: Sweet Potato and Black Bean Breakfast Burrito

Lunch: Chickpea and Spinach Quesadilla

Dinner: Vegan Sweet Potato Chickpea Curry

Snack: Roasted Edamame with Sea Salt and Pepper

Sunday

Breakfast: Berry and Nut Oatmeal

Lunch: Roasted Vegetable and Hummus Wrap

Dinner: Zucchini Noodles with Pesto

Snack: Avocado and Tomato Salad

Week 5

Monday:

Breakfast: Blueberry Almond Overnight Oats

Lunch: Caprese Salad with Balsamic Glaze

Dinner: Mushroom and Lentil Shepherd's Pie

Snack: Cheese and Whole-Grain Crackers

Tuesday:

Breakfast: Sweet Potato and Black Bean Breakfast Burrito

Lunch: Chickpea and Spinach Quesadilla

Dinner: Vegan Sweet Potato Chickpea Curry

Snack: Cucumber and Avocado Salsa

Wednesday:

Breakfast: Berry and Nut Oatmeal

Lunch: Roasted Vegetable and Hummus Wrap

Dinner: Zucchini Noodles with Pesto

Snack: Avocado and Tomato Salad

Thursday:

Breakfast: Greek Yogurt Parfait

Lunch: Lentil and Vegetable Soup

Dinner: Stuffed Bell Pepper with Quinoa and Black Beans

Snack: Roasted Chickpeas

Friday:

Breakfast: Blueberry Almond Overnight Oats

Lunch: Spinach and Feta Stuffed Bell Peppers

Dinner: Mushroom and Spinach Lasagna

Snack: Greek Yogurt and Berry Parfait

Saturday:

Breakfast: Avocado Toast with Tomato

Lunch: Mediterranean Chickpea Salad

Dinner: Vegan Sweet Potato Chickpea Curry

Snack: Hummus and Veggie Sticks

Sunday:

Breakfast: Berry and Nut Oatmeal

Lunch: Caprese Salad with Balsamic Glaze

Dinner: Cauliflower Fried Rice

Snack: Trail Mix with Nuts and Dried Fruits

Conclusion

If you're yearning for swift, health-conscious, and mouthwatering vegetarian meals, "Vegetarian Dash Diets Cookbook" is your ultimate solution. Having embraced these recipes, you now hold the key to crafting your culinary delights. Feel empowered to adjust ingredients, adding your personal touch to every dish. Soon, you'll not only have crowd-pleasing recipes but also cherished favorites for your private indulgence. This cookbook unlocks a world of possibilities, ensuring you meet your dietary goals without compromising on flavor. Savor the journey to a healthier, more flavorful lifestyle!

Author's afterthought

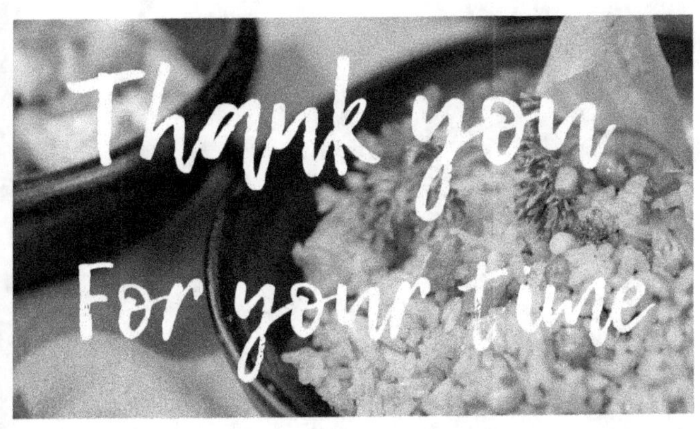

A heartfelt thank you to you my cherished reader who took the time to delve into "Vegetarian Dash Diets Cookbook"!

Amidst numerous choices, you chose this book, and for that, I extend immense gratitude. Whether you found joy in these pages or discovered valuable insights, I have a small favor to ask. If you could spare a few minutes to share an honest and heartfelt review on **Amazon.com**, your support would be invaluable. Your reviews make a significant difference and contribute to helping others benefit from this book.

Thanks again for being part of this journey!

www.ingramcontent.com/pod-product-compliance
Lightning Source LLC
Chambersburg PA
CBHW070850260726
48661CB00004B/1333